ETHICAL DEBATES

The Debate About
Genetic Engineering

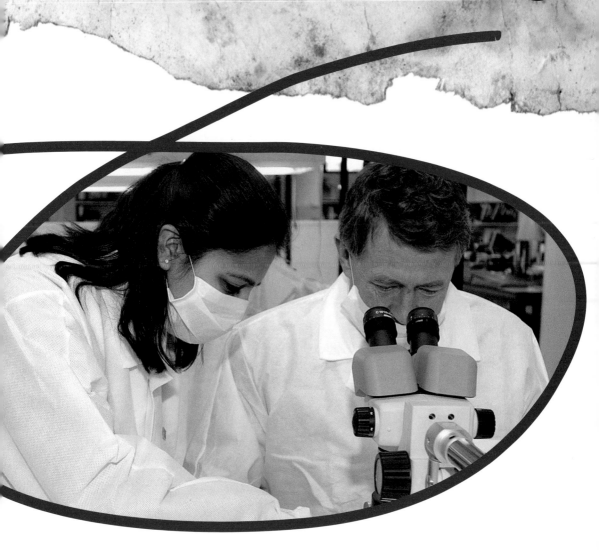

PETE MOORE

rosen publishing's
rosen
central

Published in 2008 by The Rosen Publishing Group, Inc.
29 East 21st Street, New York, NY 10010

First Edition
Editor: Patience Coster
Series Editor: Camilla Lloyd
Consultant: Dr. Jane Freedman
Designer: Rita Storey
Picture Researcher: Diana Morris

Picture acknowledgments: AP/Topham: 39 Tony Arruza/Corbis: 11. Jacek Bednarczyk/epa/Corbis:
41. Bettmann/Corbis: 6. Dr. Jeremy Burgess/Science Photo Library: 37. CC Studio/Science Photo
Library: front cover, 45. CDC/PHIL/Corbis: 9. Jack K Clark/Image Works/Topfoto: 21. CNRI/Science
Photo Library: 16. Jim Craigmyle/Corbis: 33. Dodds/Topfoto: 22. Eye of Science/Science Photo
Library: 20. Mauro Fermariello/Science Photo Library: 25. Christopher Fitzgerald/Image
Works/Topfoto: 28, 30. Jon Freeman/Rex Features: 29. Grace/zefa/Corbis: 24. Tom Grill/Corbis: 8.

Steve Gschmeissner/Science Photo Library: 17. Christina Koci Hernandez/SF Chronicle/Corbis: 43.
James King Holmes/Science Photo Library: 10. H. Huber/U. Starke/zefa/Corbis: 14. Makoto
Iwafuji/Science Photo Library: 13. Jeff J. Mitchell/Reuters/Corbis: 5. Larry Mulvehill/Image
Works/Topfoto: 27. Oak Ridge National Laboratory/US Dept of Energy/Science Photo Library: 38.
Dr. M. Ottabert, Pitie-Salpetriere, ISM/Science Photo Library: 44. PA/Topham: 32, 35. Alfred
Pasieka/Science Photo Library: 34. Picturepoint/Topham: 7. Reuters/Corbis: 36. J. C. Revy/Science
Photo Library: 19. St. Bartholomew's Hospital/Science Photo Library: 18. Sipa Press/Rex Features:
42. Steve Warmowski/Journal-Courier/Image Works/Topfoto: 12. Lee Jae-Wonj/Reuters/Corbis: 31.
Library of Congress Cataloging-in-Publication Data
Moore, Pete.

Library of Congress Cataloging-in-Publication Data

The debate about Genetic engineering / Pete Moore. -- 1st ed.
    p. cm.
Includes index.
ISBN-13: 978-1-4042-3754-4 (library binding)
ISBN-10: 1-4042-3754-2 (library binding)
1. Genetic engineering--Moral and ethical aspects. I. Title.
QH438.7.M663 2007
660.6'5--dc22
                              2006100305

Manufactured in China

contents

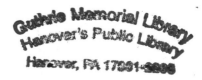

Headline hitters

This case study highlights some of the issues that surround the debate on genetic engineering.

case study

Headline hitters

In spring 1997 the world heard with amazement that Dolly the sheep had been born. Dolly was an ordinary sheep who had been brought to life by an extraordinary process. Animals normally start life when a sperm from the father comes into contact with an egg from the mother. The genes in the sperm combine with those in the egg. This process of sexual reproduction creates a unique set of genes and brings a new, unique individual into being.

In the case of Dolly, this did not happen. Instead, scientists took a cell from the udder of a six-year-old ewe (female sheep). They placed this next to an egg that had had almost all of its genes removed. The scientists then sent a short pulse of electricity through the cell and the empty egg, causing them to combine and start growing. Amazingly, the cell and egg started to develop into an embryo (see page 26). Unlike normal embryos that have genes from two different adults (the mother and the father), this embryo had all its genes from one sheep—the six-year-old female. This process is called "cloning." Dolly was a clone of the six-year-old ewe. The public and most scientists were stunned.

Why the fuss? Although most people did not know it, there was nothing new about cloning. Scientists had been cloning amphibians, like frogs, for years. They had also cloned mammals in the first few days after sperm and egg joined to form an embryo. What was new with Dolly was that they had taken a cell from an *adult* mammal and generated a new individual.

This raised the possibility that scientists could clone an adult human. It also made the world think about the different uses of genetic technology. Many people started asking whether it was acceptable to use all of the powerful techniques, or whether some of them should be banned. Before Dolly, most people had not given much thought to the discoveries that scientists were making. After Dolly, they started to ask questions. Some people are excited by the new possibilities, others feel that the more they find out about genetic technology the more worried they become.

It's a fact

A gene is a piece of biological information stored inside cells and passed on to future generations. Genes instruct cells how to perform a specific action. Many genes tell cells how to build specific proteins.

▼ Two children look at the preserved remains of Dolly the sheep—the world's first mammal cloned from an adult cell—as she goes on display at the National Museum of Scotland in Edinburgh. Dolly, who was born on July 5, 1996 after her creation by the Roslin Institute research center, died in February 2003 after the decision was taken to "euthanaze" her when it was discovered she had a progressive lung disease.

It's a fact

In the world of science, there is always a delay between scientists finishing an experiment and the results being made public. In the case of Dolly, the sheep was actually born on July 5, 1996, and she was nine months old before most people had heard about her. This time delay gives fellow scientists the opportunity to check whether the research has been done properly.

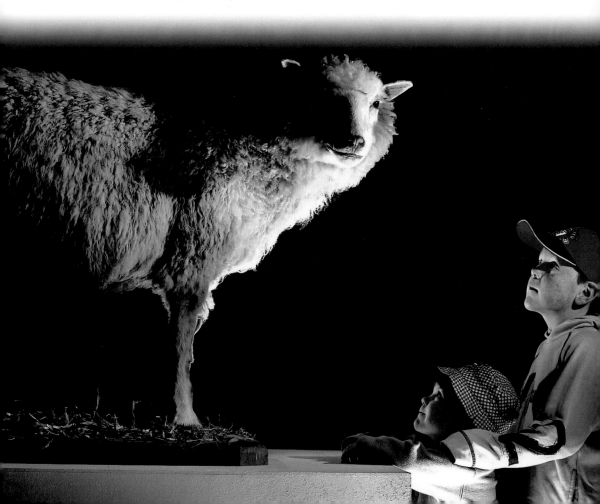

CHAPTER 1

From genius to genes

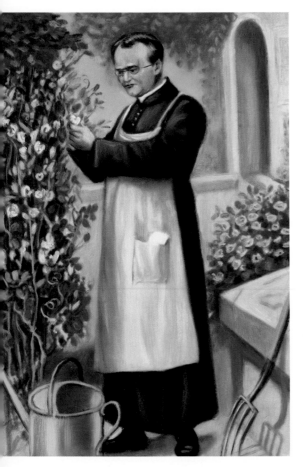

▲ Gregor Mendel works away quietly in the gardens of an Austrian monastery. His carefully performed experiments were an important step in the understanding of genes and genetics.

Modern genetics can be traced back to a quiet-mannered Austrian monk called Gregor Mendel, who was born in 1822. Mendel became fascinated with the ways in which plants inherit different characteristics, for example, the shape of peas or the color of flowers. He grew plants, pollinating them carefully so he knew which parent plants had given rise to which new plants. He monitored the way in which their shapes and colors passed through the generations.

The experiments were complex, but by 1866 Mendel had come to some important conclusions. He realized that some physical element must be passed on from parents that enabled their offspring to inherit features such as flower color or pea shape. He also spotted that different features such as pea shape and color were inherited separately and were not linked—the inheritance of flower color, for example, is not linked to the inheritance of seed shape.

Cell structure and DNA

Over the next few decades, other scientists came to similar conclusions. The next question to answer was: where was this information stored? Living organisms are made up of cells, and scientists realized that each cell needed to contain a full copy of all this information. Organisms grow when cells grow and divide into two. Each of these two new cells needs to have a complete copy of the information. For this to happen, the cells need a mecanism by which they can copy the information and put it in each new cell.

It's a fact

Not all the DNA in cells is contained in the nucleus. A small amount of DNA is also found in cells in small "packages" called mitochondria.

During the twentieth century, scientists came to realize that this information was stored in the cell nucleus. They discovered that the material in the nucleus that was most likely to enable the copying of information was a molecule called deoxyribose nucleic acid—DNA.

It was not easy, however, to understand how DNA could store information and pass new copies of it into new cells. Speculation ended in 1953 when the scientists Francis Crick and James Watson announced that they had discovered DNA's structure. They showed that the molecule consisted of two strands that wound around each other. The strands were linked together by four different sets of atoms, called bases, that scientists write down as A, T, C, and G. Crick and Watson realized that these four bases could spell out a code sequence. Also, the way in which the two strands linked together gave clues to how the information could be copied.

By carefully studying cells through microscopes the scientists saw that the DNA was gathered together into 46 separate dumbbell-shaped clumps. Because these clumps could easily be dyed they were called "chromosomes"—the Latin word for "colored bodies."

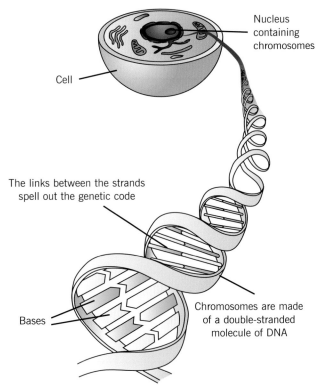

Nucleus containing chromosomes

Cell

The links between the strands spell out the genetic code

Bases

Chromosomes are made of a double-stranded molecule of DNA

▲ This diagram shows what DNA would look like if one of the chromosomes was stretched from the nucleus of a cell.

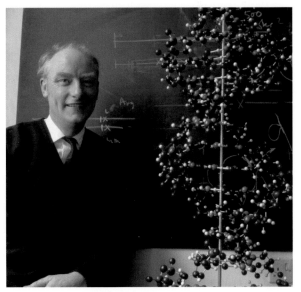

▲ Francis Crick, one of the people who discovered the structure of DNA, shown here with a model of the DNA molecule.

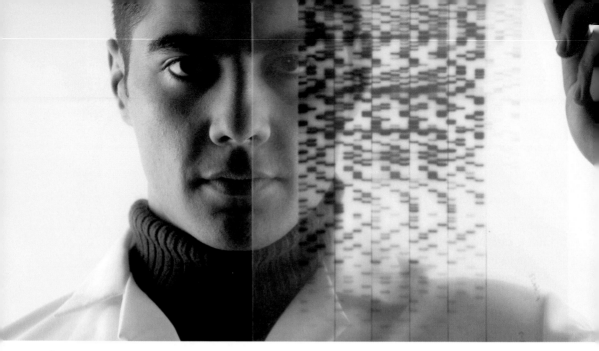

▲ One stage in finding the sequence of bases in a genome creates a sheet of dots. A computer scanner can then turn this into useful information.

The human genome

Once scientists knew the basic structure of DNA, they focused on discovering how cells manage to use this information. In the 1960s, various scientists found that the four different bases act like "letters" in a four-letter alphabet. In humans, the information is stored in 3 billion bases. That is the equivalent of more than 6,000 standard paperback books. This full set of information is often called the genetic code—scientists call it the human genome.

The genetic code is surprisingly simple. In English, or any other written language, information is stored by arranging letters in the right sequence. Cells do exactly the same thing. Their genetic code is created by arranging the four bases in a specific sequence.

Late in the 1960s, scientists found that some viruses contain molecules that act like "genetic scissors." They called them restriction enzymes. These scissors cut

DNA at very specific sequences of bases. By using these scissors, scientists started to find out where individual genes were within the genetic code. They then found that they could cut a gene out and discover its sequence of bases.

A single gene can contain many thousands of bases. As scientists studied genes, it became clear that in some cases changing just one base stopped the gene from working. Some genes are so important, that if they stop working the cell is damaged. Then, the plant or animal may develop a disease, known as a "genetic disease," because it is caused by a faulty gene. On occasion, however, a small change in the genetic code will produce a gene that creates a slightly different or improved effect within a cell. This is how chance mutations allow organisms to evolve.

A common language

As geneticists looked at different plants and animals, something became clear. The same basic molecule, DNA, carried information in every life form. It was there in bacteria, plants, mice, and humans.

This stimulated a new area of work. A gene sequence that produces a specific protein in one organism will still produce that protein if it is inserted into another. For example, genes that create certain human proteins needed in different medical treatments have been placed in bacteria. The bacteria then create the protein. This is a cheap way of growing a medical therapy.

▼ Finding the sequence of bases in DNA takes years of careful laboratory work. The sequences of many animals, plants, bacteria, and viruses are now known.

The discovery of genetic engineering meant that scientists could identify individual instructions within the genetic code, read the sequence of bases, see what happened when they changed one or more of the bases, and move the sequence into new organisms. The question is, just because it is possible to manipulate living things in this way, is it always right to do it?

summary

▶ Genetic engineering refers to a wide range of techniques that enable scientists to influence the genes in individual cells or whole organisms.

▶ Cloning is one of the more extreme examples of genetic engineering.

▶ Information is stored inside cells on chromosomes.

▶ The information-carrying part of chromosomes is made of DNA.

▶ DNA contains a sequence of code built with four different bases named A, C, G, and T.

▶ The exact sequence of these bases spells out the cell's instructions.

▶ In genetic engineering, scientists read and manipulate this sequence.

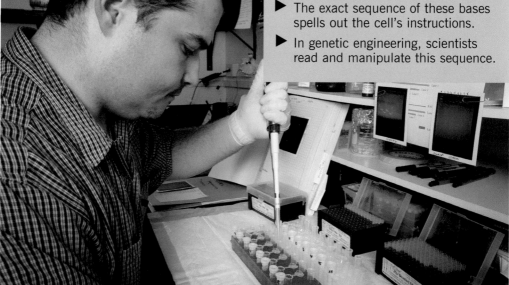

CHAPTER 2

Agriculture

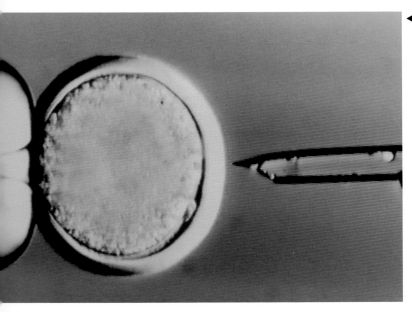

In some forms of genetic engineering, a sperm can be injected directly into an egg. Here scientists hold a spherical egg still by sucking it onto the tip of a very thin tube. They then use a tiny glass needle to puncture the egg and inject a single sperm.

Farmers keep animals so that people can either eat something the animal produces, such as milk or eggs, or eat the animal itself. Over the centuries, farmers have selected animals that have different useful characteristics and bred them with one another. This has produced breeds of sheep, cattle, pigs, and poultry that now meet specific needs. For example, some breeds of cattle, such as black-and-white Friesian cows, produce a lot of milk but very little meat. Other breeds, such as the black-haired Aberdeen Angus, produce little milk but substantial amounts of meat.

Breeding and genetics

These breeding programs take many years to produce results but, now that much more is known about genetics, farmers can speed up the process and make it more controlled. Genetic engineering can be used in a number of ways. One option is to insert new genes deliberately into animals. These genes may help the animal use food more efficiently, grow faster, or produce more milk.

Genetic engineering can also be used to monitor which animals carry which genes. Using this information, breeders can set up breeding programs that deliberately select specific features in a much more precise way. Although the animals have not been genetically modified, genetic technology has played an important role in their breeding.

In traditional breeding programs, the breeder selects animals whose characteristics he or she wants to see in the next generation. Then the breeder puts two animals—a male and a female—together and waits for them to mate.

If the animals are, for example, dairy cattle then the breeder has to wait for around nine months for a calf to be born, then a further couple of years before the female calves can give birth and start producing milk. This means it takes almost three years before a breeder of dairy cattle can discover whether the selective mating has produced a useful calf.

Now, however, breeders can take sperm and eggs from male and female animals and create an embryo in a laboratory dish. They can then take one cell from the embryo and analyze the genes in it. This will show which embryos are most likely to carry the features the breeders hope to see in the next generation. The breeders select the embryos they want, place them in the wombs of female cows, and allow them to develop. The unwanted embryos are destroyed. This process makes breeding programs faster and more successful.

Intensive farming—benefit or harm?

Breeding programs have revolutionized agriculture. They have resulted in cows that produce ten times more milk than

▼ Intensive farming: over several decades, selective breeding programs have reduced the time it takes for chickens to grow to full size from around 12 weeks to 6 weeks. Genetic engineering could create similar changes in much less time.

nonintensively bred cows. This gives the consumer high volumes of milk at low prices. But the stress placed on the cow means that she frequently suffers from infections in her udders and has difficulty walking. As a result, farmers sell these cows for low-grade meat when they are only six or seven years old. Nonintensively bred cows may live up to 25 years.

In less economically developed countries (LEDCs), scientists are tracking down the genes that enable cattle to withstand high temperatures or live on small amounts of water. This could lead to breeding programmes that give poor farmers in LEDCs access to cattle that are better at surviving drought. But how can poor farmers afford to pay for this research?

It's a fact

Chickens farmed for their meat have now been bred so that they grow to full size within six weeks of hatching. While this means they can be produced cheaply, it also results in them having weak bones that break easily, and the intensive housing conditions can lead to the rapid spread of disease.

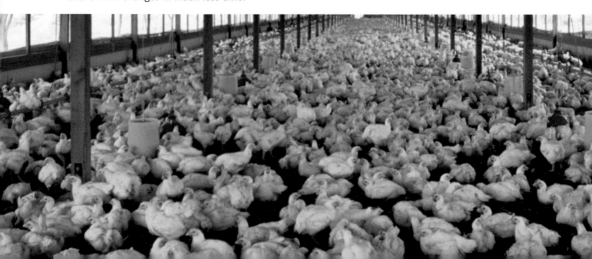

Modified farm animals

Genetic engineering opens up many possibilities for the future. One possibility is to alter the genes in animals. This is called genetic modification (GM). It is possible, for example, to add an extra growth hormone gene to farm animals. Growth hormone is a molecule that an animal produces. This hormone travels around in the animal's blood, controlling many aspects of the way in which it grows. Scientists have performed experiments in which they have added extra copies of this gene to sheep. The scientists found that the modified sheep could grow taller and faster. They also produced twice the amount of milk and grew more wool than ordinary sheep.

So far the problem is that the animals with the extra gene require more looking after than ordinary sheep. They may grow taller,

but they tend to be thinner and are at a greater risk of developing diabetes. Their hooves grow faster and require more frequent clipping.

▼ A vet injects cattle with a growth hormone at a U.S. livestock market. A small amount of hormone is put in the ear of most cattle after they have been auctioned. This means that farmers end up with animals that grow faster.

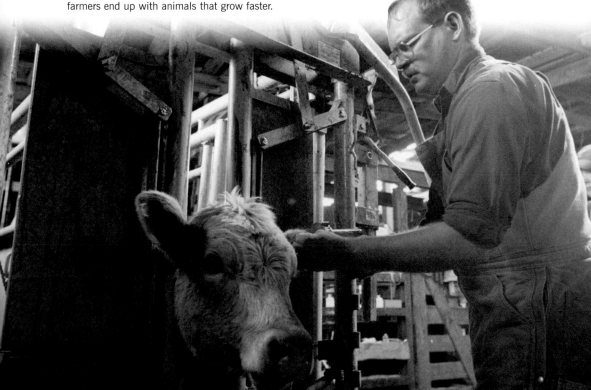

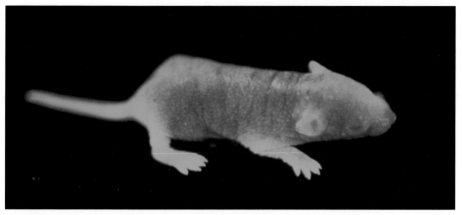

▲ Scientists want to develop ways of moving genes from one animal to another, but sometimes they find it difficult to see whether this transfer has worked. One way of checking is to practice with a gene that can make cells glow in ultraviolet light, as with the mouse above.

From farming to pharming

Another possibility is the altering of animals so that they do something slightly new. Farmers keep animals because they are an efficient way of turning plant crops (for example, grass, which animals eat) into different forms of protein (milk, which humans drink, and eggs and meat, which humans eat). It is now possible to add new genes to animals like sheep and goats to make these modified animals produce new proteins in their milk. A few animals have been modified to produce medical drugs in their milk, and some chickens to generate unusual proteins in their eggs. It is then relatively simple to collect the milk or eggs and purify the protein.

In one situation, a gene has been added to sheep, which causes them to produce spider-web silk in their milk. This silk can be harvested and woven into incredibly strong ropes or lightweight stab-proof vests for human use. While these modified animals may produce useful materials, some people question whether it is ethical to turn animals into factories. Other people say that normal agriculture already does exactly this—it uses animals to transform plant matter into milk, meat, eggs, and leather.

case study

Supersize fish

Aqua Bounty Technologies is a genetic engineering company based in Massachusetts. It has created a salmon that grows twice as fast as a normal salmon. Ordinary salmon only grow in strong sunlight, because exposure to the light switches on their growth hormone gene. The scientists at Aqua Bounty have replaced the genetic mechanism that controls the growth hormone with one taken from another species of fish, the ocean pout, which needs less light to grow. These modified salmon now grow all the time.

The scientists claim that these genetically modified fish will cost less to grow, but will look and taste just like normal salmon. However, even if the fish are safe to eat there are concerns about the effect they could have if they escaped into the wild. The fear is that these modified fish would grow more rapidly and use up all the available food, so that the natural fish would die out.

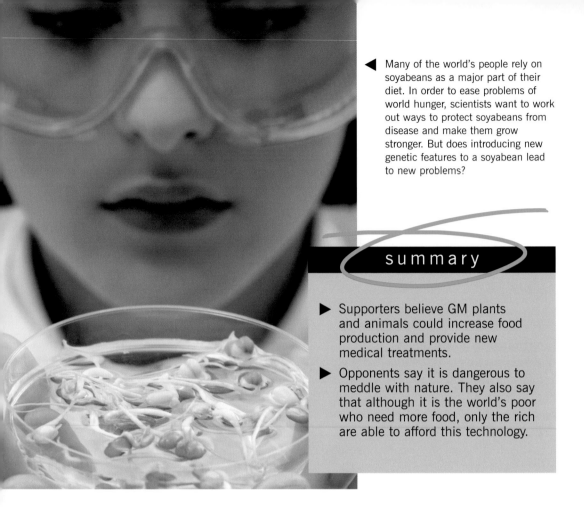

Many of the world's people rely on soyabeans as a major part of their diet. In order to ease problems of world hunger, scientists want to work out ways to protect soyabeans from disease and make them grow stronger. But does introducing new genetic features to a soyabean lead to new problems?

summary

▶ Supporters believe GM plants and animals could increase food production and provide new medical treatments.

▶ Opponents say it is dangerous to meddle with nature. They also say that although it is the world's poor who need more food, only the rich are able to afford this technology.

GM crops

Only a few genetically modified crops are grown commercially, but they cover millions of acres of land around the world. Most modifications aim to protect crops from insect pests or weeds. This is important. Insects alone destroy around 25 percent of the world's food, enough to feed one billion people—one-sixth of the world's population. The need for food will also become more urgent because the world's population is expected to increase to at least nine billion by 2050.

The most widely grown crop is "Round-up Ready" soy. This type of soy has been genetically modified to resist Round-up, a weedkiller that destroys almost all other plants. In 2002, more than 50 percent of the world's soybeans came from GM crops. Supporters of GM crops say that they are simpler and less expensive to grow. Before planting normal soy, farmers clear the weeds by plowing; they also spray them with weedkillers. During the crops' growing season, the farmers spray them with more weedkillers to keep the weeds down. This process takes a lot of time, as well as large amounts of chemicals and diesel to fuel the spraying machines.

Round-up Ready soy simplifies the process. Farmers plant the beans and let the crop and weeds grow. Then they use a single spray of Round-up. This kills everything in the field except the Round-up resistant soy. As the soy plants are already established, very little light reaches the soil so new weeds cannot start growing. The field therefore stays free of weeds. The farmer saves time and money and does not need to spray as many chemicals.

Another GM crop, *Bt*-maize, now occupies 30 million acres of the world's land. Scientists have inserted a gene from the bacterium *Bacillus thuringiensis* into *Bt*-maize, which makes the plant produce a protein that kills insect pests like the cornborer insect. Farmers do not need to spray insecticide on this GM crop.

Are GM crops safe?

What risks, if any, are involved when GM products enter the food chain? In the case of GM canola plant grown to produce cooking oil, the dangers appear to be slight. With GM canola, the oil is squeezed from the seed. All of the genetically modified material is left in the plant and none goes into the oil. The oil is exactly the same as oil from normal canola. It is difficult to see how using this oil can pose any danger. But the leftover plant material is fed to farm animals. Could these animals be put at risk? With soybeans and corn, the modified material does go into food. Some people ask whether the new protein could do

harm, for instance, by triggering food allergies. Others argue that millions of people eat the products each day in the U.S. and there is no evidence of harm.

What effect do GM crops have on the environment? Crops with builtin insect-killing chemicals do reduce the numbers of insects in an area. This means the number of insect-eating birds in the area will also be fewer. But is that a problem?

Making a profit

Many farmers, especially those in poor countries, do not sell all of the grain or beans they grow. Instead they keep some back so they can sow them and produce the next year's crop. However, companies that create GM crops need to recover the money they spend on research. Not only do they need to recover the money spent, they also must make a profit. The companies do this by making farmers buy new seed each year. They argue that the farmers benefit because new seeds tend to give bigger crops and higher yields. But opponents of this practice say the farmers cannot afford this, and that the system is unfair because it involves poor farmers sending money to fund rich businesses.

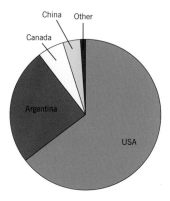

▲ Ninety-nine percent of all the world's genetically modified crops are grown in four countries.

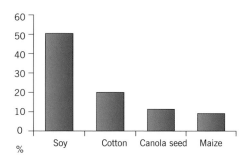

▲ The four most common genetically modified crops in terms of their percentage of the world's GM harvest.

CHAPTER 3

Medicine

Genetic engineering is increasingly being used in the field of medicine. One area of medical care that is being transformed by genetic technology is cancer therapy. In 2005, around 58 million people died in the world, and about 7.6 million of these deaths were from cancer. Over the last two decades, the detection and treatment of many forms of cancer has improved. This is largely because scientists have discovered which genes normally protect a cell from cancer, and what happens when these genes "go wrong."

▼ Breast cancer kills half a million women a year around the world. This magnified image shows healthy breast cells, but if genes in them become damaged the cells can form tumors.

It's a fact

People often talk about a cancer gene, or a gene for a particular disorder. In most cases, the gene is one that builds a protein needed by the cell for healthy living. Problems start when an error occurs in the gene and it becomes mutated.

This mutated gene then creates a faulty protein, which causes a disorder to develop in the body.

BRCA1 and BRCA2 are often called breast-cancer genes. Usually the BRCA gene makes a protein that protects a person from cancer. But when the gene has mutation 1 or mutation 2, the protein stops working properly and the person loses her protection. Her chance of contracting cancer therefore increases.

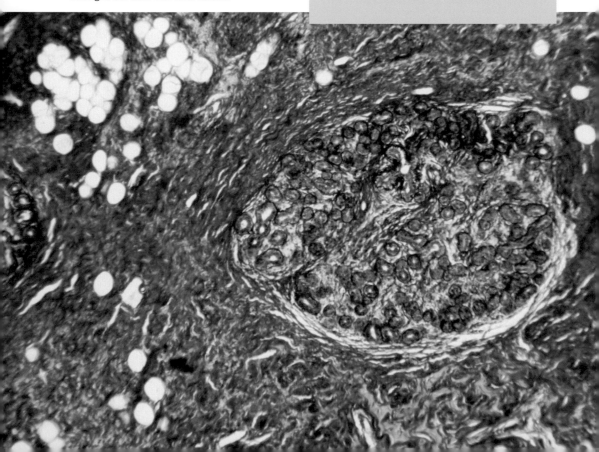

Cancer cells

Healthy cells in the body grow, split into two, then pause before growing any more. This enables the body to grow or to repair damaged or worn-out tissue. Once the cells have grown enough, they stop. Cancer occurs when a cell is out of control. Cells grow and divide without pausing. These diseased cells invade organs in the body and prevent them from working properly. If the diseased cells are not removed by a surgeon or killed by cancer treatments, they can cause serious illness or death.

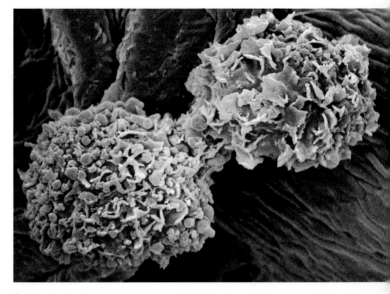

▲ This magnified image shows breast cancer cells which have not responded to signals that normally tell cells to stop growing. Instead, they have multiplied rapidly, forming a tumor.

Many different genes keep each cell under control. Some genes create proteins that monitor whether a cell is healthy or damaged. Others regulate the time at which a cell can grow and split into two. These genes work together so that only healthy cells are allowed to grow. Unhealthy cells either pause while they repair themselves or self-destruct if the damage is too severe. Cancer occurs when a series of errors builds up in the genes that control this monitoring and growth. Scientists believe that a cell needs to have errors in at least 12 of these genes before it becomes out of control.

One difficulty of treating cancer is that of finding a drug that will kill the cancer cells but leave the healthy cells unharmed. By studying the genetics of cancer, scientists are discovering specific differences in cancer cells. Chemists are able to target these differences with new drugs.

Laboratory animals

Many scientists say that we can only understand how genes work in cancer by experimenting on animals. The most commonly used animal in cancer research is the mouse, and hundreds of thousands are bred and used in research each year. Many of these mice have been altered by genetic engineering. Some have had their genes modified so that they develop particular types of cancer. Others have been modified so that they are ideal animals for testing particular types of drug.

Scientists opposed to using animals in research are developing ways of gathering information from cells grown in test-tubes. Scientists who use animals in research say that this work will always be limited, because cells developed in this way behave very differently from the way animal cells behave. Cancer research must therefore balance the benefit it gives to humans with the harm it inflicts on animals.

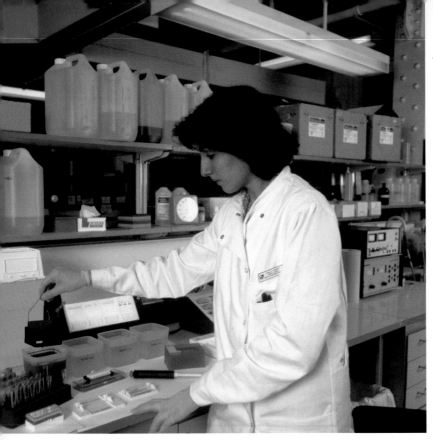

◀ Screening tests can quickly show whether or not a person is carrying a gene that could cause diseases, such as sickle cell anemia. However, if a person is told this information, what can he or she do about it?

Health screening

While genetic engineering is changing the treatments doctors offer, it is also creating tests that can reveal the chance of a person getting a specific disease in the future. These "screening tests" look for changes in genes that scientists now know are linked to particular disorders.

Huntington's chorea is a disease that starts when a fault occurs in a single gene. The gene produces a protein needed by the brain; if the gene is not working properly the sufferer experiences memory loss, aggressive behavior, and loss of muscle control. The symptoms only start when a person is aged between 30 and 50, and there is no cure for the disease. Before showing the symptoms, people with Huntington's chorea live perfectly normal lives.

Huntington's chorea is passed on from parent to child. If a person has one parent with the disease, he or she will have a 50:50 risk of suffering from it as well. Children who watched their parents struggle with the disease used to have to live with the knowledge that they might well contract it in the future.

It is now possible to have a screening test for the faulty gene. Genetic engineering means that doctors can see if the Huntington gene carries the particular fault. People can find out whether they are clear of the disease, or whether it will hit them in the future.

In a few years, doctors will be able to run a series of genetic tests on babies soon after birth. These tests will reveal the chance of the babies developing disorders like colon cancer, Huntington's chorea, or possibly,

Alzheimer's disease later in life. The tests might also show doctors which drugs are likely to help, and which could cause harmful side-effects.

Do people really want this information? They may like the idea of a doctor knowing how to treat them more effectively; and, if the test shows that a person does not have the gene, then the worry is removed. However, does a child really want to know that he or she has a high risk of developing a disorder later in life—especially if there is no cure? There are also possible future problems: an employer may think twice about giving a person a job if that person is likely to become ill; and health insurance will be harder to obtain if there is evidence that a person will develop diseases such as Huntington's chorea.

▼ This pattern of bars comes from a screening test for cystic fibrosis, and can show whether a particular fault is present.

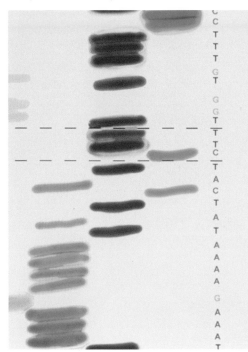

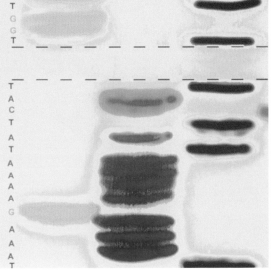

case study

Who do I tell?

Jane is 50 years old and has just had a genetic screening test. The results show that she has a high risk of developing breast cancer. To reduce the risk of getting cancer, she decides to have an operation to remove her breasts. Jane has two daughters aged 20 and 24, and a sister aged 57. Their close relationship to Jane means that they have a high chance of sharing this gene. Should she tell them about the results of her test, so that they can get tested as well?

She decides to tell them. The daughters are pleased to know; they have the test. One daughter shares the gene mutation and has the operation to remove her breasts. The other does not have the gene, and starts to feel guilty that she does not need the operation. Jane's sister is furious. She says she did not want to know about this risk, and that she will never talk to her sister again. She also blames Jane for upsetting her daughters.

Gene therapy

Many diseases are caused when bacteria or viruses enter a person's body and stop cells from working properly. Other diseases occur because one of the body's own systems is not working properly. The reason for this is that one or more of the body's genes carries faulty information.

There are currently around 4,500 different known diseases that occur when just one gene is damaged. The most common are cystic fibrosis (see page 24), sickle-cell anemia and x-linked hemophilia. The person has the disease because a faulty gene is building a protein molecule that is the wrong shape and cannot work properly. Scientists hope that by introducing a new copy of the gene that carries the proper code-sequence, they can enable the body to produce working versions of the protein. They call this treatment gene therapy. Doctors first attempted gene therapy in 1990. The hope that gene therapy will succeed is still there, but so far no fully safe treatment has been developed that has a long-term cure.

Curing future ills?

Most forms of gene therapy place new genes in the body's cells. The treatment tries to avoid the new genes being placed

▼ Healthy red blood cells are disk-shaped with a dip in the middle. People with sickle-cell anemia produce misshapen red blood cells (below) that carry oxygen less efficiently than healthy red blood cells.

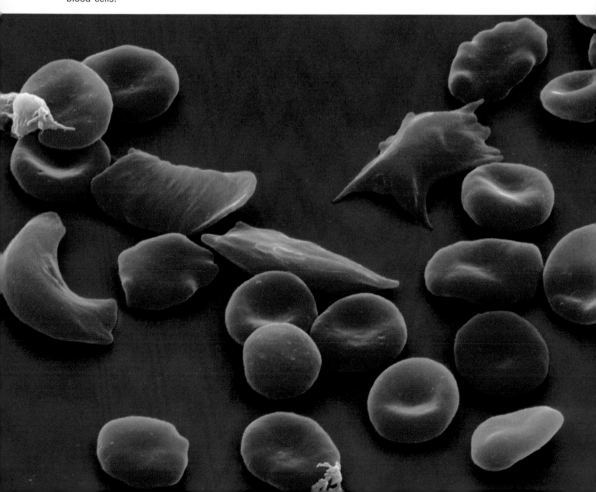

in cells that form eggs and sperm. This way, the new genes cannot be passed on to future generations. The treatment, and its risks, are limited to one person.

Some people say that if gene therapy can eradicate a disease, we have a moral duty to place it in sperm and eggs. This could stop future generations of people from suffering from the disorder. But adding the gene to these cells means that it will be present in the person's children and grandchildren. How certain do we need to be that the process is safe before we use such a permanent form of therapy?

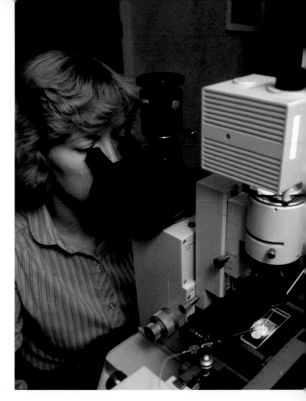

Inserting genes into cells requires highly ▶ technical equipment.

case study

A risk worth taking?

In the year 2000, doctors in Paris, France, started using a treatment on 11 children who were suffering from an illness which meant they could not fight diseases. They therefore had to live in isolation bubbles to avoid contact with bacteria and viruses. The cause of the children's disorder was a faulty gene that prevented their bone marrow from producing white blood cells to fight infection.

The doctors inserted long needles into the middle of the children's leg bones and removed some of the bone marrow. They then took some viruses and placed a working version of the bone marrow gene in the virus. The doctors mixed the bone marrow cells with these modified viruses. The viruses infected the bone marrow cells and placed the gene inside the cells. This new gene enabled the bone marrow cells to start

producing healthy, white blood cells. The bone marrow was then placed back in the patients and their bodies were soon able to start fighting infection.

Two years later, two of the children developed a form of leukemia—a cancer that affects blood. It appears that this had been triggered by the viruses that carried the new gene into the bone marrow. Nine of the children had been helped and remained in good health. All of the children survived, but they would probably have died without the treatment.

The experience of the children raises a number of questions. When it is safe to start using a new treatment? Should a treatment be given if most patients benefit, even though some could be harmed? What is an acceptable level of risk?

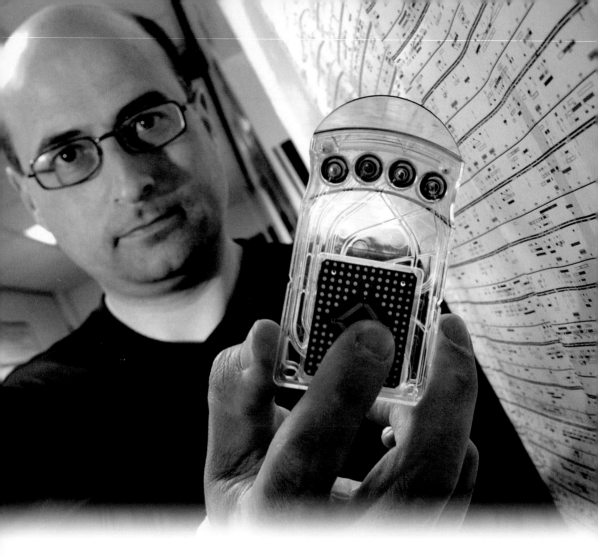

▲ Professor Peter Ghazal of the Scottish Centre for Geonomic Technology and Information holds a microchip of the human genome in his hand.

The human genome

Inside almost every human cell is a nucleus. This nucleus contains most of the cell's DNA, packaged into 46 chromosomes. DNA is a ladderlike molecule in which the rungs are made up of four bases. Information is stored in DNA by arranging these four bases in a specific order—just as information is contained in a sentence by arranging letters and spaces in a specific order. The full set of information is contained in 3 billion bases and it is called the human genome.

It's a fact

Humans have about 25,000 genes. Mice have about 30,000 genes. Ninety-nine percent of human genes are present in mice. This is one reason why mice are such useful animals in medical research.

In 1988 a group of scientists at Cold Spring Harbor Laboratories near New York, came up with an ambitious plan. They decided that it was technically possible to determine the full sequence of bases in the human genome. If the project was to be completed in any sensible timeframe, however, it would require a huge financial investment and hundreds of scientists and technicians.

The project started with 42 scientists working in 17 countries. A year later, theteam had grown to include 220 scientists in 23 countries. By the end of the project, more than 1,000 people were working on it. The aim was to complete the work, which cost around $200 million a year, within 15 years. It was the largest single biological research project ever attempted.

When they started, few people realized that laboratories would soon be full of inexpensive personal computers. This new computing power enabled the scientists working on the Human Genome Project to race ahead. By the year 2000, they had worked out the vast majority of the sequence—three years ahead of schedule. Since then, the genomes of other species have been written down. This means scientists can now compare the human sequence with sequences taken from many living things, including mice, chimpanzees, and many bacteria and viruses.

Not everyone is happy with the Human Genome Project. Critics complain that while vast sums of money have been poured into sorting out the genome, other areas of research have been starved of funds. Researchers working on practical projects that could immediately help poor people say that their funding has been reduced and channeled into a project that will largely help the rich.

viewpoints

"Let us be in no doubt about what we are witnessing today—a revolution in medical science whose implications far surpass even the discovery of antibiotics."
British Prime Minister Tony Blair, speaking in the year 2000

"Mapping the human genome is a great human achievement, rather like climbing Mount Everest. Like climbing Mount Everest, it will benefit few people, leaving most untouched. But unlike climbing Mount Everest, it has the potential to damage large numbers of people."
Dr. Richard Nicholson, editor of *Bulletin of Medical Ethics*

summary

▶ Supporters say increased knowledge about human genetics may lead to new ways of finding out why people are ill and predicting whether they may become ill in the future. It can also be used to develop new ways to treat sick people.

▶ Opponents say people do not always want to know if they will become ill in the future, and that the new treatments are costly and potentially dangerous.

CHAPTER 4

Designing babies

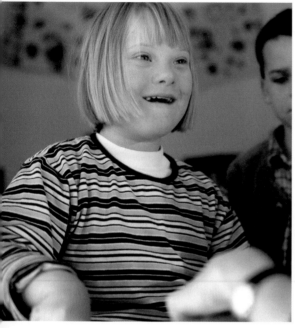

▲ People with Down's Syndrome have an extra chromosome, which can be detected while babies are still in the womb. But what should parents do if they are given this information about their unborn child?

Every month scientists develop more genetic tests to tell if people are likely to suffer from a specific disease. When people discover that they have one of these faulty genes, they are faced with a number of choices. In some cases they may look for treatment that makes the disease less damaging, or in other cases they can alter their lifestyle.

One decision they will have to make is whether or not to have children. If a person has a disease-linked gene, there is a possibility that he or she could pass this on. Many people want to have children, but do not want to pass on the disease.

case study

A difficult decision

Susan and Guy have been living together for five years. They have decided that they would like to have a baby. Both of them, however, have close family members with cystic fibrosis. This disease affects many parts of the body, it is very painful and debilitating and many sufferers do not live for more than 30 years.

Cystic fibrosis is caused by a fault in one gene. Each person has two copies of this gene. If only one copy is damaged, the person will be healthy, but he or she is a "carrier" of the disease and the faulty gene can pass to his or her children. If a person has two damaged genes, he or she has the disease.

If both partners are carriers, there is a one-in-four chance that any child they have will be born with two damaged genes and will have the disease. Susan and Guy both take a genetic test and find that they are carriers. They have various options. They can split up and find new partners who have been screened and know they are not carriers. They can have a child and accept the one-in-four risk that it will have cystic fibrosis. They can use medically assisted reproduction to create an embryo that can be tested for the disease before it is placed in Susan's womb. Or Susan can get pregnant and have the fetus tested. At this point, she and Guy can decide whether or not to continue with the pregnancy.

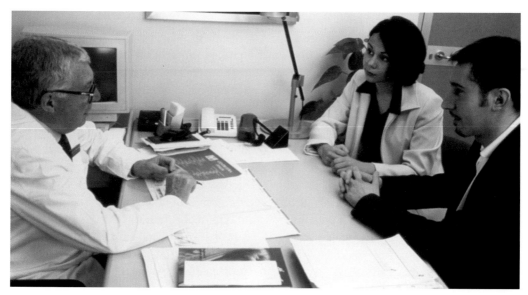

▲ About one in ten couples has problems
conceiving a baby. Genetic technology is
introducing many new options for such couples.

Playing God?

A combination of genetic engineering and
medical technology now offers a new
solution. Doctors can bring a couple's
sperm and eggs together in a laboratory to
create an embryo. After a few days, the
embryo will have grown so that it consists
of around eight cells. Scientists can remove
one of the cells and test its genes. If the
test shows that the disease-linked gene is
in the cell then the scientists discard the
embryo. If the test shows that the gene is
not in the cell, then the embryo is placed
in the woman's womb and allowed to
develop. This process is called pre-
implantation genetic diagnosis.

However, some people are concerned that
scientists who use this method may be
"playing God," by actively seeking to
remove genetic disorders from our society.
These people think that this is a kind of
eugenics—the despised form of
population control that was practiced in
some parts of the USA in the early part
of the twentieth century, and in Nazi
Germany in the 1930s and 1940s.

Also, once we allow screening for severe
genetic diseases, where do we stop?
Should this test be used to screen and
avoid a mild mental illness, for example?
Should we allow screening to look for
genes that may influence attention span, or
for genes linked to sporting ability?

In most cases, the tests will be performed
on embryos. Some people, who believe
that embryos are full human beings say
that this is a form of murder. Others argue
that the desire to reduce the risk of
children being born with disabilities
discriminates against disabled people.
Those people who want screening to be
carried out say that we should try to
prevent new people with disabilities
coming into existence, while at the same
time we should also look after existing
people who have disabilities.

Sex selection

One use of genetic technology is to enable parents to decide whether their next baby will be a boy or a girl. There are two main reasons why parents might want to choose the sex of their baby.

Firstly, there are medical reasons. Several hundred inherited diseases only affect boys. If people know they are carrying a form of gene that causes one of these diseases, they can avoid having a child with the disease by selecting to have only girls. Secondly, there are non-medical reasons. Parents who already have a boy may want to 'balance' their family by having a girl. Also, in some cultures boys are more

valued than girls. This may be because boys can earn more money than girls. In some countries, such as India, parents of girls must pay a dowry to the groom's family when their daughters marry. This payment may cripple a poor family financially, so sex selection is often used to try to have boys rather than girls.

Many people are unhappy with the idea of choosing any features of future children. They say that it turns the child into a commodity, much like a designer item that can be bought in a store. But those in favor of sex selection say that it "adds value" because parents are more likely to cherish a child they really want.

◀ At fertilization, a sperm combines with an egg. If the sperm contains an X chromosome, the embryo will end up with two X chromosomes and develop into a girl (fig. a). If the sperm contains a Y chromosome, the embryo will have one X and one Y chromosome and develop into a boy (fig. b).

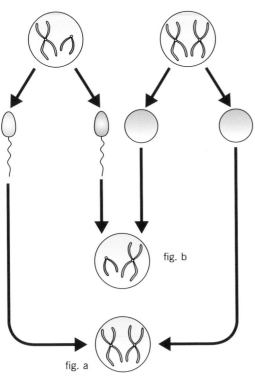

fig. b

fig. a

It's a fact

A person's sex is determined by two of their 46 chromosomes. These two chromosomes are called the sex chromosomes. There are two types of sex chromosome, an X and a Y. A person with two X chromosomes will be female. A person with one X and one Y chromosome will be male. When sperm and eggs develop they each contain only one sex chromosome. Women's cells have two X and no Y chromosomes, so their eggs can only have an X chromosome. Men's cells have an X and a Y chromosome, so their sperm can contain either.

Methods of sex selection

A single sperm carries 23 chromosomes. One of these will either be an X or a Y chromosome (see box on page 26). The X chromosomes are larger than the Y chromosomes, so sperm carrying X chromosomes are marginally heavier. Scientists can use this difference in weight to separate X and Y sperm. The system is not perfect, but using sorted sperm can greatly increase a couple's chance of choosing their child's sex.

Another option is to bring sperm and eggs together in a laboratory dish. After fertilization, the embryo grows for a few days and the doctors remove one of its cells. This cell can be tested to see if it has a Y chromosome. If it does, it is male—if it does not, it is female. Only embryos of the chosen sex are placed in the woman's womb.

If a woman conceives naturally, then a baby starts to grow in her womb. After a couple of months, the fetus is big enough for doctors to use ultrasound scans to determine its sex. The woman may then be able to seek an abortion if the baby is not of the desired sex. In the UK, abortion is not allowed for sex selection alone, but it is possible to abort a boy fetus if it means that the mother can avoid having a child with a specific sex-linked disease.

▼ A hospital technician performs an ultrasound scan on a pregnant woman.

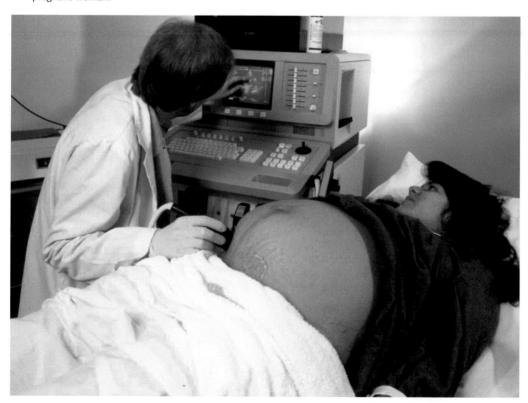

Donors

Some diseases destroy organs or stop them from working properly and the only option is to try to replace them. If the heart or kidney needs replacing, doctors transplant an organ from a person who has just died. In some cases, the person with the disease does not need to receive whole organs. Many different diseases are caused when a person's bone marrow stops working properly. Doctors sometimes treat these patients with drugs that kill all the bone marrow cells, and then inject new healthy cells from a donor. The donor only needs to give a small sample of cells, because these will then multiply once they have been injected into the patient.

The problem with this treatment is that human bodies have immune systems that kill any new cells entering them from outside. The immune system mainly kills bacteria and viruses, but it could also attack donor cells. Doctors therefore need to find a donor with cells that are so genetically similar to the patient's that his or her body does not kill them. Brothers, sisters and other close relatives are the most likely people to share similar genes, but doctors often cannot find a donor.

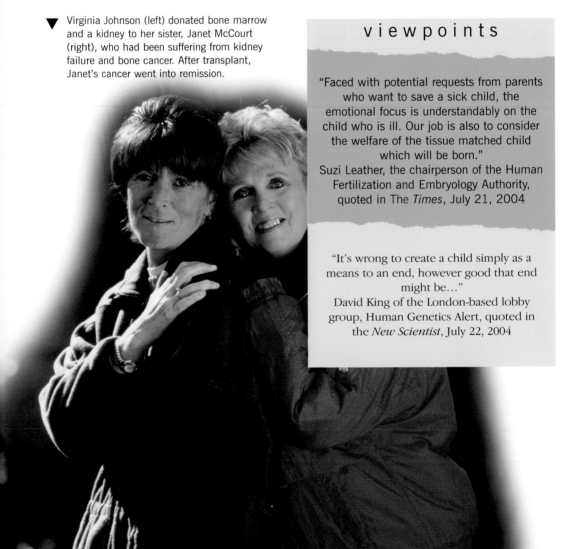

▼ Virginia Johnson (left) donated bone marrow and a kidney to her sister, Janet McCourt (right), who had been suffering from kidney failure and bone cancer. After transplant, Janet's cancer went into remission.

viewpoints

"Faced with potential requests from parents who want to save a sick child, the emotional focus is understandably on the child who is ill. Our job is also to consider the welfare of the tissue matched child which will be born."
Suzi Leather, the chairperson of the Human Fertilization and Embryology Authority, quoted in The *Times*, July 21, 2004

"It's wrong to create a child simply as a means to an end, however good that end might be…"
David King of the London-based lobby group, Human Genetics Alert, quoted in the *New Scientist*, July 22, 2004

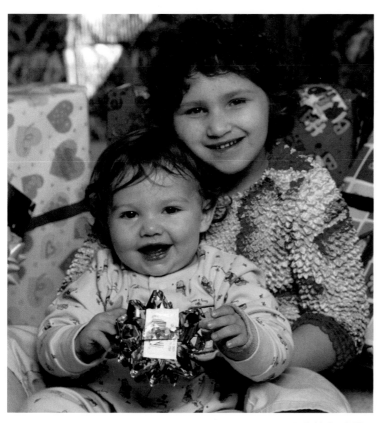

◄ Molly Nash, who suffers from the rare blood disease, Fanconi anemia, with Adam, her baby brother. Adam was genetically engineered so that cells from his umbilical cord could be used to boost Molly's immune system.

Savior siblings

The solution then may be to take some eggs from the patient's mother and sperm from the patient's father and use them to create embryos in a laboratory. These embryos have a strong chance of possessing the same sort of genes as the patient. Using methods developed by genetic engineering, each of these embryos can then be tested to look for the one that is the best match. When doctors find a suitable embryo, they place it in the mother's womb and let it develop. When the baby is born, doctors collect cells from the umbilical cord and donate them to the sick person.

But is it right to bring a new baby into the world purely for the purposes of helping another child? Many people say that the new child is being used to create a medical treatment. Others are worried that many embryos will be created and destroyed before a matching one is found. They say that this devalues human embryos.

It's a fact

The first so-called savior sibling was born in the USA in the year 2000. Adam Nash was born after doctors had selected an embryo with the same tissue type as his sister, Mollie. She had a rare but fatal condition, recessively inherited Fanconi anemia. While the treatment helped Mollie, doctors destroyed 30 embryos before they found the one that became Adam.

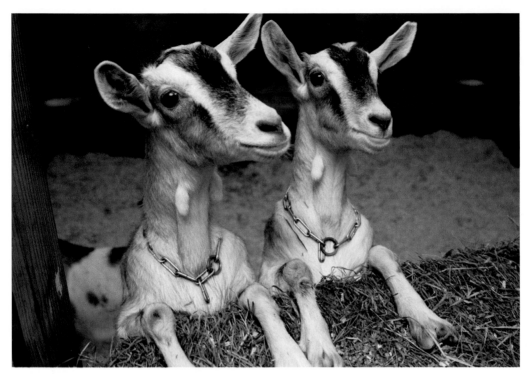

▲ Cloned goats in Massachusetts: while most attempts at cloning are unsuccessful, scientists have managed successfully to clone sheep, goats, cows, mice, pigs, cats, and rabbits.

Cloning

Dolly the sheep proved that cloning mammals was possible, but she also demonstrated that it was very unsafe to try it in humans. To begin with, the research team that produced Dolly took 277 attempts before they achieved one successful pregnancy. In the years that followed, the success rate only improved a little. Also, most sheep that are kept in ideal living conditions live for between 11 and 16 years, but Dolly was killed humanely when she was only six years old because she was developing disorders that are normally found in old sheep. One reason that scientists gave to explain Dolly's ill health was that the cell used to clone her had been taken from an adult animal and somehow "remembered" its age. This meant that when Dolly was born, her cells thought she was already six years old. Throughout an animal's life its cells pick up genetic errors, so it is quite possible that Dolly had started life with an error-filled cell.

Creating a replica

One of the reasons people may want to create a clone is to have a replica of someone who already exists. But how closely will this clone match the person who donated the cell? While clones share many physical similarities, they will have their own individual set of experiences, which will strongly influence their characters. And what would it be like to grow up knowing you are someone's clone? Would other people be able to treat you as a unique individual? Would you feel free to be you?

Therapeutic cloning

Another use of cloning does not aim to create a new individual, but to make genetically identical cells and maybe even organs. In the same way scientists created Dolly, doctors could take a cell from a patient and fuse it with a human egg that had had its nucleus removed. They would then send an electrical pulse through these cells to stimulate them to start developing into an embryo. At this point, any of the embryo's cells has the possibility of growing into any organ in the body. Scientists are developing ways of guiding the cell's development so that they can make specific types of cells.

This "therapeutic cloning" has the potential to solve many serious diseases. In 2005, a team in South Korea announced that they had cloned human cells. This would have been a major breakthrough, but later in the year the work was shown to have been faked.

Opponents of therapeutic cloning say that the process will be very difficult to control, and the new cells might easily turn into cancer tumors. They are also concerned that it will be necessary to create an embryonic clone in order to treat a patient. This clone will then be destroyed to generate the new cells.

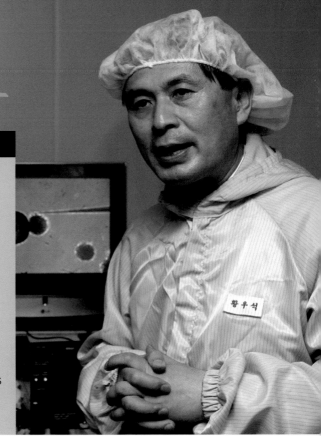

► Hwang Woo Suk, leader of the team of South Korean scientists who falsely claimed to have cloned human cells.

summary

- ► People in favor of genetic engineering believe that it can provide new ways to prevent the next generation of children inheriting serious genetic diseases.
- ► People who oppose it believe screening embryos is a new form of eugenics, and will lead to screening for other features such as characteristics linked to intelligence or sporting ability.
- ► Opponents also argue that screening devalues human embryos and turns babies into commodities.

CHAPTER 5

Forensics and crime scenes

Genetic engineering is now being used to solve crimes such as bank fraud, robbery, assault, and murder. Police try to track down criminals by looking for things they have left behind at a crime scene, including pieces of body tissue containing their DNA.

Police and their forensics teams look for obvious items, like blood, but they can collect DNA from saliva (for example, if the criminal has licked an envelope before mailing a letter), strands of hair, and pieces of nail, skin, and bone. DNA may also be found on the rim of a wineglass, where a person was drinking from it, and on the discarded butt of a cigarette.

When police look at DNA they usually do not concern themselves with genes because these do not vary much from one individual to another. In between the genes, however, are long sequences of DNA, which do vary greatly between individuals. As a result of genetic engineering there are now tests that can quickly record the unique features of these sequences of DNA. The results of these tests are known as a genetic fingerprint. The forensics team also look for Y chromosomes to determine whether a cell has come from a man or a woman. On occasions they can use certain gene tests to discover the racial origins of the person who left the cells behind.

▼ A police forensics team at work gathering evidence at a murder scene in Dublin, Ireland.

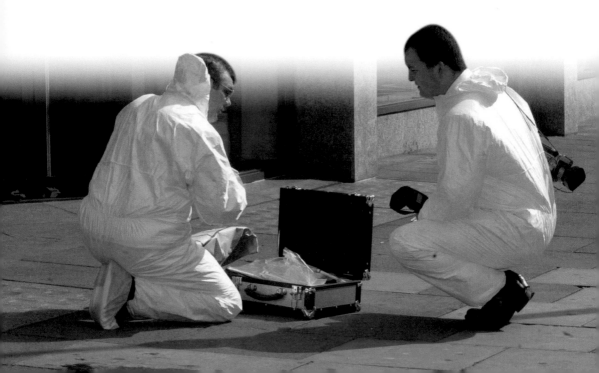

case study

Edward Honaker

Defense lawyers often use DNA evidence to prove that a person is innocent. For example, in 1984 an American man called Edward Honaker was convicted of attacking and sexually assaulting seven different people. He was given three life sentences. He always protested his innocence and was able to provide witnesses who confirmed that he was somewhere else at the time of the attacks.

After a few years in prison, Honaker contacted an organization that works to free wrongfully convicted people. They tested his DNA and the DNA found on some of the victims' clothing. The two were very different. These tests proved that Honaker could not have been the attacker. He was released from jail in 1994.

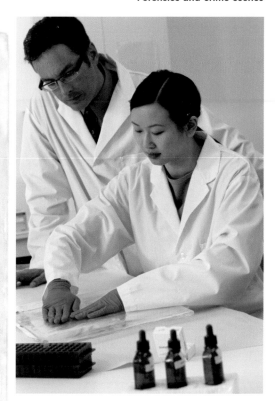

▲ Forensic scientists testing for saliva.

Three strengths

Genetic technology provides police with incredibly powerful tools. Firstly, a person's genetic fingerprint is unlikely to be found in anyone else. Secondly, scientists have developed ways of multiplying the DNA inside cells. If the forensics team recovers a sample as small as a nail clipping or a strand of hair, they can isolate the DNA, duplicate it, and then analyze it. Thirdly, DNA survives remarkably well. The DNA in a spot of blood can be analyzed weeks, months, and sometimes, years after it has been deposited.

Weaknesses

Even if the DNA found at a crime scene appears to match a sample that police collect from a suspect, there is still a remote chance that this match could have occurred by chance. After all, scientists know that members of the same family share very similar genetic fingerprints. Also, a match does not prove that the person committed the crime. For example, an innocent person may leave a strand of hair on a bus seat and that hair may get stuck to another person's jacket. This person then commits a crime and the hair falls off and is later found by the police. All of a sudden, the innocent person has become a suspect. DNA can be found in such small samples that it is theoretically easy for a criminal to deliberately "set someone up" by leaving traces of someone else's DNA behind.

A full set of male human chromosomes arranged in their pairs. The pair at the bottom right are the sex chromosomes. The X is the larger and the Y is the smaller.

UK criminal database

In April 1995, the UK government set up the National DNA Database, run by the Forensic Science Service. By 2006, the database had more than three million records of individual people's DNA, making it the largest DNA database in the world. On 45 percent of occasions when DNA is collected from a crime scene and loaded onto the database, it matches a record that is already held.

One reason why the database is so big is that police can take a DNA sample when they arrest someone. They can then keep this data on record permanently, even if the person is not charged for a crime, or is found innocent. While this provides a powerful crime-fighting tool for the police, many civil rights commentators feel that keeping innocent people's DNA samples infringes their right to privacy. In reply, the British Home Office says that: "People who do not go on to commit a crime have no reason to fear the retention [keeping] of this information."

It's a fact

In the UK, DNA profiles have been linked with crime scene profiles in more than 3,000 offenses, including 37 murders, 16 attempted murders, 90 cases of rape, 92 drug-related offenses, and 1,136 burglary offences.

viewpoints

"A major concern is that the police could misinterpret such DNA evidence as a *certainty*, whereas the tests can really indicate only a *probability*..."
GeneWatch, a UK public interest campaign group

"What is particularly welcome is that [genetic forensics] is as potent in eliminating those who are wrongly suspected or accused as it is in tracking down the guilty."
Lord Justice Sedley

case study

"Shoe rapist" is tracked down through DNA

In July 2006, James Lloyd was convicted of sexually assaulting six women. The conviction hit the headlines because the crimes had occurred around 20 years earlier, and Lloyd was caught after his sister had been arrested for driving a vehicle while drunk.

When Lloyd's sister was arrested, police took a sample of her cells and analyzed the DNA. They entered this data in the National DNA Database. Another group of police had re-opened the investigation into a curious set of sex crimes in which the attacker had stolen his victims' shoes. Police analyzed the DNA

from evidence collected at the time of the attacks and compared it with the records on the database.

No record matched perfectly, but there were 40 close matches. Quite possibly one of those was a relative of the attacker. One of the close matches came from Lloyd's sister. When police visited her they discovered that she had a brother who was living in the area where the attacks had taken place. After Lloyd heard that the police were asking about him, he tried unsuccessfully to take his own life. When he was arrested he admitted to having carried out the sex attacks.

▼ During a visit to the Forensic Science Service in south London, a UK government minister looks through a microscope assisted by forensic scientist Jognash Patel.

summary

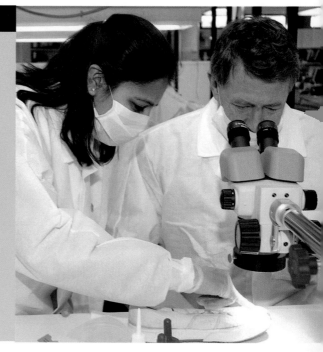

▶ Those in favor of DNA testing for evidence argue that it is a powerful way of identifying criminals.

▶ They say that genetic evidence can help prove some people's innocence.

▶ Opponents are angry that the UK's law lets police collect DNA at the time of arrest, and not when someone is charged, because they say it infringes innocent people's rights to privacy.

▶ They argue that courts need to recognize DNA data as just one piece of evidence—it is not "proof" of a person's guilt.

CHAPTER 6

The wider uses of genetic engineering

Military planners have started to look at genetic technology to see if they can use it to build weapons. They are also aware that terrorist organizations, for example, may use genetic technologies to build weapons for use against military and civilian targets, so they want to develop defenses against these weapons.

Germ warfare

Scientists can modify deadly, disease-causing microbes and select genes that enhance their ability to infect people. If released into the population, infectious bacteria and viruses would spread very quickly and cause maximum harm. It would be very difficult to contain the outbreak, and the disease could soon spread to the people who had launched it in the first place. This means that such weapons would probably only be used by terrorist organizations, who fight by creating fear.

A more remote possibility is the development of chemical or biological weapons that target a particular racial group. The underlying theory to this is that closely related people share similar patterns of variations in their genes. This means that members of a specific group of people will have particular strengths and weaknesses. It is theoretically possible to develop a drug, or maybe grow a bacterium that could specifically attack this weakness.

▼ U.S. soldiers wear gas masks as they take part in a chemical, biological, and radiological warfare exercise in Yonchon, South Korea, in February 2003. There are fears that genetic engineering could be used to enhance the effects of chemical and biological weapons.

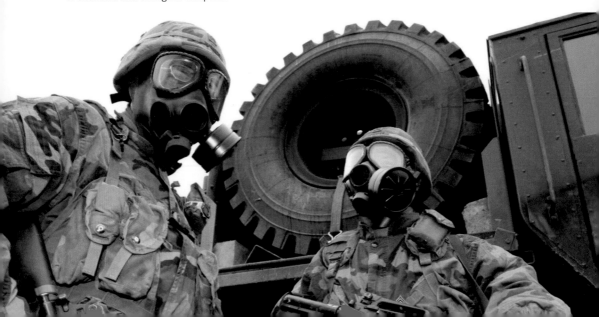

Thale cress can be genetically ▶
modified so that its leaves change
color if it grows over an
unexploded landmine.

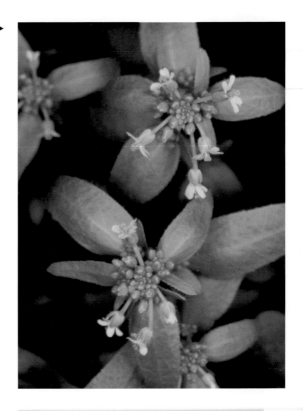

Genetic engineering can also be used to help protect against enemies who use biological agents. For example, the American Centers for Disease Control is trying to modify the smallpox virus. Its aim is to be in a better position to develop vaccines against the virus in case a terrorist organization releases it in a biological attack.

Landmine-detecting plants

More than 100 million landmines are buried around the world. Landmines are small bombs that explode when someone treads on them or drives a vehicle over them. Military planners use them to create "no-go" areas. They cost only a few dollars to make, but more than a thousand dollars to detect and destroy. At current rates of clear-up, it will take until around the year 3100 to remove all the mines that have been laid so far.

Scientists in Denmark have modified the plant Thale cress (*Arabidopsis thaliana*) by adding to it a gene that can detect unexploded bombs. Explosive devices give off nitrogen dioxide gas. The plants are green, but produce a red pigment in the fall. The genetic modification makes nitrogen dioxide switch on the red pigment, so that any plants growing over unexploded mines will have red leaves. The researchers have also modified the plants so that they need an unusual fertilizer in order to grow. This should prevent them from spreading. The problem is that if there is a cheap and effective way of clearing landmines then armies may be encouraged to use more of them.

v i e w p o i n t s

"A decade ago, the WHO [World Health Organization] was planning to destroy the world's last remaining samples [of smallpox]. Today, it is proposing to tinker with the virus in ways that could produce an even more lethal smallpox strain. This is a devastating step backward [for humankind]…"
Sujatha Byravan, executive director of the Council for Responsible Genetics

"[Using plants to detect landmines] is a pioneering example of how we will see genetically engineered plants applied for humanitarian and environmental purposes in the future."
Professor John Mundy, University of Copenhagen

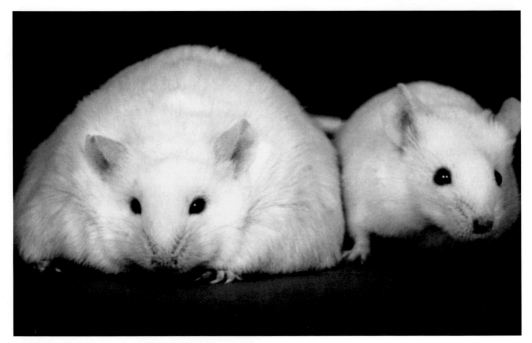

▲ A few laboratory mice have been given extra copies of the growth hormone gene. The result is a "mighty mouse" much larger than normal. But are these sorts of experiments ethical?

Sports

When people take part in competitive sports a lot is done to keep the competition fair. In power sports, such as boxing or weight-lifting, men and women do not compete against each other because male hormones tend to make the men naturally stronger. In school sports, competitors are also grouped by age. The idea is that the winner is the person who tries hardest and uses his or her skills most successfully.

Genetics, however, is starting to change things. Scientists can now analyze an individual's gene mutations for a reasonable indication of whether he or she will be good at endurance sports or sprinting. Such a test enables people to select sports in which they are likely to be successful. Although they will obviously still need to train hard, they can use the data from the genetic test to make an informed decision about their choice of sport. But critics fear that some people might use genetic tests such as this to gain an unfair advantage.

A more common fear is that people will boost their performance by injecting themselves with human hormones. One currently banned hormone is erythropoietin (EPO). This boosts endurance by increasing the number of red blood cells in the blood. In 1985, scientists found the gene that makes EPO and placed a copy of the gene in bacteria. These bacteria now pump out EPO. Sports people can get away with injecting small amounts of this type of EPO because it is the same as the hormone they already have in their bloodstream. Injecting extra amounts simply boosts the level. They would only be found out if they injected too much and the level of EPO rose far above normal values.

Another fear is that, in the future, sports people will use a form of gene therapy to place genes such as the EPO gene in their muscles. At the moment this is not technically possible, but if it ever became so it would be very difficult to detect. Scientists who have placed extra copies of the gene that makes certain growth-stimulating hormones in mice and rats have discovered that this can radically increase the animal's strength and stamina. The process also prevents muscles from becoming weaker in old age.

Some commentators believe it is impossible to stop athletes and sports people using genetic techniques. They say that two categories of fair competition should be set up—one for ordinary people and one for people who have been "genetically enhanced."

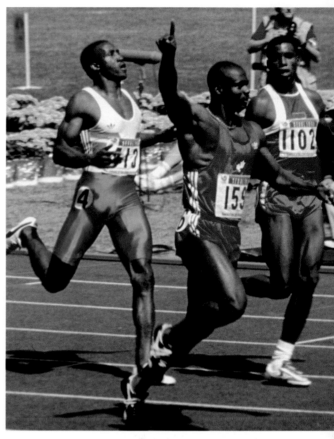

▲ Performance enhanced: athlete Ben Johnson wins the 100-meter dash at the 1988 Seoul Olympics. He was later disqualified because he tested positive for drug use and, in 1989, confessed to using steroids.

v i e w p o i n t s

"You would have to be blind not to see that the next generation of doping will be genetic…"
Dick Pound, the chairman of the World Anti-Doping Agency, the organization that checks whether athletes use illegal drugs

"If it's not dangerous, [gene doping should not be banned], it just levels the playing field…"
Ron Clarke, Australian elite athlete

s u m m a r y

▶ Genetic technology raises many new possibilities in areas as varied as warfare and sport.

▶ These new possibilities will need new systems of regulation to prevent them from doing more harm than good.

CHAPTER 7

Finance and the future

Patents have existed since at least the fifteenth century. A patent is a legal way for inventors to register their inventions. They can then prevent other people from using them. Alternatively, inventors can let people use them, but charge them for doing so. If inventors are unable to register a patent, they may want to keep their work secret. A patent protects a person's idea for twenty years. When patents work well, they encourage people to come up with new ideas and share them with others.

Patenting life

Until 1980, no one was allowed to patent any life form because such things were considered to be part of nature. However, in 1980 a court case in the U.S. Supreme Court effectively changed the rules. Since then, many patents have been given to people who have discovered the sequence of genes. This has given biotechnology companies a chance to make a profit from the money they invested in the research that revealed the gene.

Some people do not think it is right that a person can claim ownership over genetic material at all. In regular types of patent, the invention must be new. This cannot be the case for genes that have been around for millions of years. Opponents of this practice ask: how can a person claim to have invented a gene sequence when it has been present in millions of living organisms for millions of years? Supporters of patenting say that DNA is not "life," and therefore patenting it raises no ethical problems.

Regular types of patent must usually involve an inventive step. In the case of most genetics patents, no inventive stage takes place, although some geneticists claim that the ways of making use of the gene sequence sometimes involve a form of invention. Also, anything that is considered to be a "discovery" is not generally eligible for patenting. Many people think that finding the sequence of a gene is a discovery, not an invention.

Opponents of genetics patenting are particularly annoyed when people are given patents for modified animals. Canada is the only industrialized country not to give patents for "higher life forms" such as genetically modified mice. One problem with gene patents is that companies use them to stop competitors from working on certain genes. This takes away any competition and slows down the rate at which scientists come up with new ideas. It also stops other scientists from developing alternative ways of using the gene.

It's a fact

In genetics patents, inventors must:
identify new genetic sequences;
specify what the sequence will produce in a cell;
specify the product's purpose—in other words, say what it does in a cell;
enable an expert to use the sequence for its stated purpose.

viewpoints

"To our minds, the risks of [gene] patents far outweigh the potential benefits, and they should be prohibited…"
Mildred Cho, associate director at the Stanford University Center for Biomedical Ethics and associate professor of pediatrics (genetics)

"Intellectual property protection [patents] for gene-based inventions will play an important role in stimulating the development of important new healthcare products…It's quite simply a case of no patent, no cure…"
Andrew Sheard, chairman of the Bioindustry Association's intellectual property advisory committee

▼ Professor Zdzislaw Smorag (left) and doctor Maria Skrzyszowska (right) from the Zootechnical Institute at Krakow in Poland present a rabbit born as a result of a new method of somatic cloning. The method is awaiting patenting. The scientists hope the new procedure will be useful for raising animals to produce proteins for pharmaceutical use and for modifying animal organs for possible human transplantation.

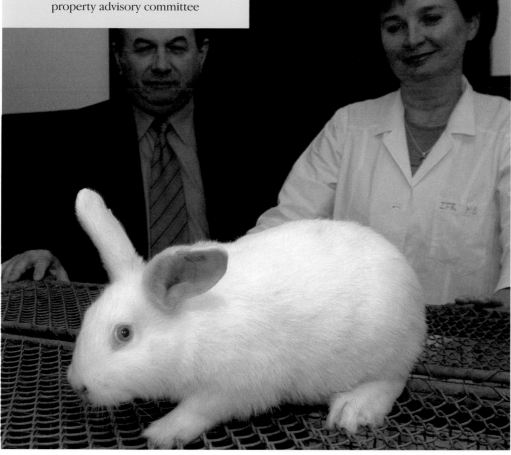

Insurance

One fear that most people have is that something will happen to them that either prevents them from earning money or will be costly to resolve. For example, their house may catch fire, leaving them with a huge repair bill, or their kidneys may stop working properly, meaning that they can no longer go to work.

One way of preparing for if the worst should happen is to take out an insurance policy. In effect this means that a large number of people join a kind of club where they all make a small, regular contribution to a central fund. This fund will then pay out large amounts of money to the few people who need it in difficult times.

For the insurance process to work, it is necessary for the members of the "club" each to pay a fair amount into the central fund. A member who poses a high risk will be asked to pay more than a low-risk member. For example, males under the age of 25 pay high insurance fees if they want to drive a car. This is because they run a higher risk of being involved in an accident than women of the same age or older men. They pay more because, in the event of an accident, they are more likely to ask for money from the insurance company.

When people take out insurance policies that pay out if they are ill, they must warn the insurance company beforehand if they have had, or still have, health problems. The company then calculates the person's risk of getting sick, and sets a fair rate of payment. This system only works if the people and the insurance company have access to the same information.

Asking genetic questions

People can now choose to have genetic tests that will show if they are at an unusually high risk of suffering from different types of disease, such as specific types of cancer or certain brain disorders. In most cases, the test will not show that a person will definitely be affected by the disorder. This will depend on a wide range of additional factors, including the person's diet and whether he or she smokes or takes regular exercise.

However, if a person has a faulty gene he or she knows that the risk is higher. The person may then try to take out an insurance policy, knowing that there is

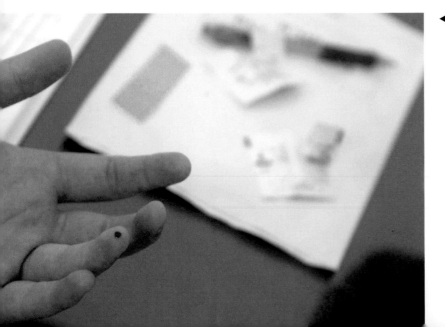

◀ A person having a blood test for a genetic disorder.

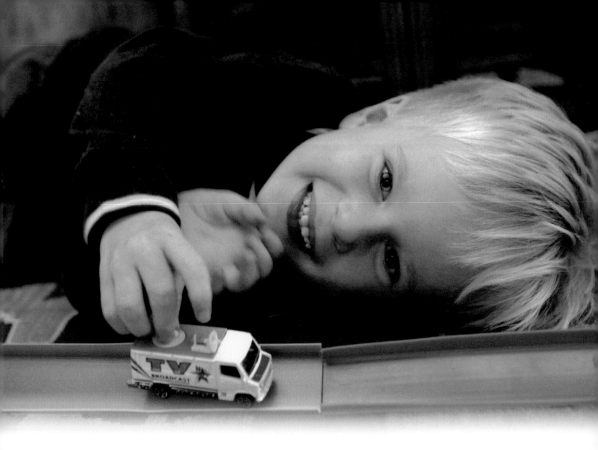

▲ In 2005 in the U.S. the parents of Jack Zembsch, a four-year-old boy with a rare bone disease, were unable to get him the treatment he needed. They accused his healthcare provider of refusing to cover his insurance for the treatment because it was too expensive. Jack's parents claimed that they were forced to meet many of his related health costs themselves.

a strong chance that he or she will ask for a large payout. If too many people do this, the insurance companies will soon pay out much more money than they take in, and the insurance system will collapse.

At the moment, insurance companies do not ask about genetic tests if a person is only applying for small levels of insurance. But there is one exception to this rule. The person must tell the insurance company if he or she has had a test for Huntington's chorea. Huntington's is unusual, because the genetic test gives a definite answer. People who have the gene for the disease will contract it by the time they reach 50 years of age. If a person is

already ill and a genetic test has helped doctors to find out what the illness is, then that person must declare the "diagnostic" information to his or her insurance company.

Genetic underclass

Many people are concerned that insurance companies will soon want to know about all genetic tests. This could make it impossible for some people to take out any form of health insurance. This would affect them in many ways. In particular people often need to have some form of health insurance before they can buy a house or take a particular job.

Future scanning

Now that scientists can read and alter genetic information in cells, they have access to a powerful technology. But where is this technology leading us, and do we really want to go there?

Scientists and doctors may use their new ability to modify genes to cure some types of disability and disease. This seems a positive step forward, until we try to define disability and disease. Clearly it would be good to cure conditions such as Huntington's chorea, which destroys nerve cells in parts of the brain. But do we want to "cure" an inability to run fast or think clearly, or a failure to grow tall? Should we try to redesign human beings to create an ideal society, or should we build a society that cares for everyone as they are?

▼ Advanced medical scanning can now detect changes in brain activity caused by genetic diseases such as Huntingdon's chorea, shown here.

In agriculture and industry, genetic engineering can create plants, animals, and bacteria capable of generating highly useful products. The task now is to find ways of sharing these benefits with many people and prevent them from simply being hoarded by the rich. Also, can we remain in control of the newly created organisms, or will they run riot and kill off other natural species of plants and animals?

summary

▶ Genetic technology is increasing people's understanding of how living organisms work.

▶ This new information enables scientists to diagnose diseases and produce new forms of treatment.

▶ The information is leading to new ways of farming crops and animals, and offers one way of feeding the growing population in the world.

▶ On the other hand, genetic technology could create modified organisms that are difficult to control.

▶ It could also lead to new forms of discrimination.

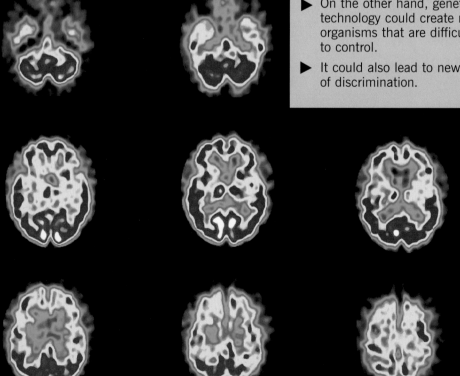

100

0

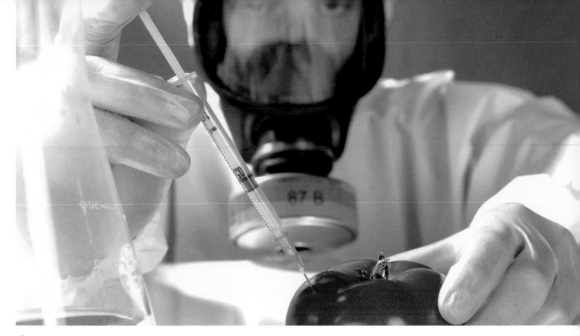

▲ It is easy to generate fear about genetic technology by misrepresenting what it involves. This pretend situation shows a person dressed in a bioprotection suit to highlight the perceived hazards of genetically modified foods.

The limits of genetics

Increasingly, scientists realize that genes do not simply dictate what goes on in cells, they play a central role in many aspects of life. However, a cell is influenced not only by its genes but also by the environment around it. For example, a cell in the body is influenced by its neighboring cells' actions as well as by its genes' instructions.

A gene is also strongly influenced by other genes in a cell. Scientists need to look at the mutations in tens or hundreds of genes before they can predict disorders more fully. In terms of genetic engineering aimed at helping humans, it is important to remember that genetic diseases are only one set of diseases. Bacteria or viruses cause many other diseases. Tests performed on an embryo to avoid some specific diseases do not guarantee that the child will be healthy. He or she could still catch some other illness; and no genetic test can prevent someone from becoming disabled in a car crash, for example.

Proceeding with care

While these debates continue, it is important to consider what is possible and what is not. For example, when scientists added a gene to rice to boost its vitamin A content, many of them claimed that this would solve nutritional problems around the world. In reality, it has made little difference. The body only absorbs the vitamin A if a person eats the rice along with green vegetables, and many of the people who need this vitamin do not have access to green vegetables.

There are many questions relating to this example. Will the people who need the vitamin A find sources of green vegetables? Will they be able to afford the modified rice? Will the modified rice have any unexpected influence on the environment? Nevertheless there is genuine hope that modifying food crops can in the future solve some nutritional problems. Genetic technology offers many benefits but, because it is such a powerful tool, we need to move forward with caution.

Glossary

Alzheimer's disease A common form of brain disease that normally only starts to occur in people over the age of 65.

Atom The basic unit of ordinary matter.

Bacterium (pl. bacteria) A form of single-cell organism; some bacteria cause diseases.

Bases The units that make up DNA. There are four different bases, and their order "spells out" the genetic code.

Bone marrow The spongy material in the center of bones that generates new blood cells.

Breeding program A system of selecting which male and female animals should mate with each other to try to create offspring with specific traits.

Chromosome The tightly packed coils of DNA inside a nucleus of a cell. Different organisms have different numbers of chromosomes, and they are often present in pairs.

Clotting factor A protein that is needed to help blood form a clot if a person or animal becomes injured. There are a dozen or so clotting factors, and if any one is missing, the individual can bleed excessively if cut.

Diabetes A disease where animals and people cannot control the amount of sugar carried in their blood.

DNA (Deoxyribose nucleic acid) A large molecule capable of carrying information that can be stored in a cell, read by it, and passed on to new cells each time the cell divides.

Embryo In mammals, a fertilized egg that is beginning to develop.

Enzyme A biological molecule that can speed up the rate of chemical reactions.

Fetus In mammals, an embryo becomes a fetus from the point at which the organs are fully developed.

Forensic From the Latin word *forensis*, meaning "of the forum." The forum was the marketplace in ancient Roman cities where authorities held court cases. The term now refers to any investigation that provides evidence that can help a court decide whether a person is guilty or innocent.

Genetic code A term used to describe the order of bases in a length of DNA.

Genome The entire sequence of DNA in an individual species.

Hemophilia An inherited disease, usually only affecting males. In hemophiliacs the blood does not clot properly and a small wound may result in fatal bleeding.

Hormone A molecule produced in one part of the body that has a controlling influence in another part.

Insulin A molecule (hormone) produced by mammals, which controls the way in which the body uses sugars.

Microbe A microscopic organism.

Molecule A group of atoms bound together in a specific shape.

Mutation The act of changing or altering.

Nucleus The compartment in a cell that contains the chromosomes.

Organism Any living animal, plant, bacterium, or virus.

Protein A large biological molecule built out of a specific set of amino acids.

Sickle cell anemia A range of diseases that occurs if people inherit faults in the genes controlling their red blood cells (the cells that transport oxygen around the body). It results in red blood cells that are the wrong shape and do not carry oxygen properly.

Sperm A single cell equipped with a tail that propels it along. It fertilizes an egg, triggering the beginning of embryonic life.

Ultrasound scan A piece of medical equipment that uses soundwaves to generate images of internal organs.

Viruses A microscopic package that can break into living cells and use the cells to produce new copies of itself.

X-linked disease A disease caused by a fault on an X chromosome. These chromosomes are passed on by mothers, but the diseases normally only affect male offspring.

Timeline

10,000 years ago Humans start selecting wild grasses and growing them together, leading to the development of modern crops, such as wheat and rice.

1859 Charles Darwin publishes *On the Origin of Species*, which focuses people's minds on the idea that information is passed from one generation to the next, and that this information will gradually alter as different individuals breed with one another.

1865 Gregor Mendel publishes the findings of his research, suggesting that biological information is held in units.

1866 Ernst Haeckel suggests that biological information is stored in the nucleus.

1869 Friedrich Miescher finds that the nucleus is packed with DNA.

1953 Francis Crick and James Watson show the way that the DNA molecule can store and duplicate information.

1968 Stewart Linn and Werner Arber discover "restriction enzymes" that exist within cells and cut DNA in specific places.

1977 Walter Gilbert and Frederick Sanger independently develop methods for determining the sequence of bases in DNA.

1990 Human Genome Project launched.

1990 First attempts at gene therapy on humans.

1996 UK government sets up the National DNA Database.

1996 Birth of Dolly—a sheep cloned from an adult cell.

2000 Draft sequence of human genome announced.

2000 The genes of an embryo are tested to identify whether or not it has a strong chance of becoming a good tissue donor for an existing child. Scientists find that it has, the embryo is allowed to develop, and a child is born as a result.

2001 Birth of ANDi, the first genetically modified primate.

2002 A religious sect (the Raelians) claim to have cloned a human, but they do not supply proof of this.

2002 DNA familial searching is used to track down a man who raped and murdered three girls in 1973.

2003 Human genome now almost completely discovered and written down.

2004 Announcement of the creation of a genetically modified plant that can identify the location of landmines.

2004 A mouse is born with two female parents and no male parent.

2004 Korean scientists claim to have taken embryonic stem cells from cloned human embryos.

2005 The Korean claim is found to be false.

Further information

Books to read:

Genetic Engineering (Cool Science series)
Ron Fridell (Lerner, 2006)

Modern Genetics: Engineering Life (Milestones in Discovery and Invention series)
Lisa Yount (Facts on File Inc., 2006)

Due to the changing nature of Internet links, The Rosen Publishing Group, Inc., has developed an online list of Web sites related to the subject of this book. This site is updated regularly. Please use this link to access the list:
www.rosenlinks.com/ed/engine/

Index